The Body Mender Cleanse

Holley B Steinberg

I would like to dedicate this book to my mother Shyrlene Byrd. If it weren't for you and what you went through, I wouldn't have created this manual. You taught me how I can help people heal by educating them on how the body works and how it can heal itself. How bitter sweet it is, that if I knew then what I know now you would still be here, but if that were the case, I wouldn't be writing this book. Thank you Mom! I really miss you, but I know you have your hand on my shoulder guiding me through this.

INTRODUCTION

I am very happy you decided to go down this path. Cleaning out your intestines and your colon is the first step in having a healthier body.

This manual will explain everything from food shopping to what to do to prepare, to what to expect during the process.

It is always recommended that you consult your doctor before you start your cleanse. Especially if you have diabetes or crones disease.

I am not a doctor, nor do I claim to be. I have done a lot of research and have learned a lot over the years I wish to share what I know to help you change and heal.

I would like to tell you about my journey and how it got me to here.

In 1999, my mother was diagnosed with rectal cancer. Because at the time, we didn't know any better, she had surgery to have her rectum removed and a colostomy bag installed. During her experience she learned about the body's pH. She taught me that when the body's pH 7.35, the body functions and heals the way it is supposed to. When the pH is 7.5, cancer will go dormant. At that time, the only thing that was available to her was coral calcium. I don't think she knew anything about food or water.

In 2005, she died. I remember one day when I was visiting (as I did daily), she grabbed my hand and said I had such healing hands. Anyone who knows me, knows I am not a touchy feely person. And why she would say such a thing was beyond me.

Two years later, I remembered what she had said, and decided to go to school to learn Massage Therapy. During my time in school, I worked for a chiropractor that offered foot detox and other alternative services. Over the last 5 years I have been able to slowly incorporate Cupping Massage, Alkaline Water and Detox Foot Baths into my business for a more rounded healing.

Many of my clients have autoimmune diseases, diabetes, IBS, constipation, etc. But one week in particular, I had a lot of people coming to me with yeast issues and constipation. Then a light bulb went off in my head and I realized if my clients would do a colon cleanse, it would help their body function better. Before we can change what we put in our body, we MUST clean our colons out.

Thanks to the help of Sylvia Anton, who wrote "The Farmaceuticals Recipes" with some great and easy recipes to go hand in hand with this cleanse. Having this book will help to keep you on track. This cleanse will change your life.

We are on this path for you!

It is recommended to read the entire manual before you start.

Chapter 1

Welcome to the Body Mender Cleanse

We live in a constipated world due to what we eat and drink or what we DON'T eat and drink. And because of this, our bodies start to shut down and stop functioning properly.

Our intestines use mucus to help slide everything through. BUT when we put something in our mouth and swallow it, the body will either decide if it is ok or NOT OK. If it is "not ok", body creates extra mucus to protect the body from the "not ok" food. When extra mucus and bad food mix together it creates a substance called "Mucoid plaque". It cakes the intestinal and colon walls to where we can no longer absorb nutrients, in fact what happens is you start reabsorbing the toxins that are in the plaque. To make things worse, the plaque gets thicker and thicker and we become more toxic.

The Body Mender Cleanse will not only IMPROVE digestion and elimination, but it will also help slow down the aging process. Suggested time for this cleanse is 10 days.

During this cleanse, you will be on a very strict diet that includes plenty of raw vegetables, juices, fruit, sprouts, salad greens, nuts and seeds with each meal. You will drink ½ of your body weight in ounces of water EVERY DAY.

Chapter 2
What to expect

During the time you are on the cleanse, you should **NOT** have:

- *Sugar* of any kind. That includes all sugar, honey, artificial sugars, and stevia. Sugar is very acidic. An overabundance of it can cause yeast (candida) to build up in the gut, which can turn into a fungus and spread. An excessive amount of yeast can cause leaky gut, which can cause autoimmune diseases in the body. We are trying to heal the gut, so sugar is not allowed.

- *Bread*. It is a carbohydrate which turns into sugar.

- *Diet soda*. With a pH of 3.2, diet soda is very acidic. They contain sodium benzoate or potassium benzoate. "These chemicals have the ability to cause severe damage to DNA in the mitochondria to the point that they totally inactivate it - they knock it out altogether," Peter Piper, a professor of molecular biology and biotechnology at the University of

Sheffield in the U.K., told a British newspaper in 1999. The preservative has also been linked to hives, asthma, and other allergic conditions, according to the Center for Science in the Public Interest.

- ***Water Flavorer's' or Flavored Water (MIO, Crystal light, Dasani, Fitness water, Vitamin Water etc.).*** They contain sugar from high fructose corn syrup, MSG (natural flavors), and **two** artificial chemical sugar substitutes - sucralose (found in Splenda) and acesulfame potassium (Ace-K)

- ***Regular Soda and Alcohol.*** Full of chemicals, carbohydrates and sugar.

- ***Processed food or fast food.*** These foods are full of calories, chemicals and have no nutritional value.

- ***Dairy.*** 1. A cow produces milk to feed her calf to grow into a 600 pound cow. 2. Whatever that cow ate or had injected into it, is going into you.

1. The first couple of days, you may experience some bloating. The fiber shake makes you full and you definitely

don't want to over eat. You could also have a headache due to your body detoxing or not having caffeine. You might be tired or sluggish. Take it easy, nap if you can. Listen to your body.

2. Your bowel should start moving on the second day. The third day, it may move A LOT!

3. This cleanse is very smooth. You should not feel as if you are going to be in the bathroom the entire time. When you do poop, you can expect it to be a large movement.

4. You could also experience the removal of "Mucoid Plaque". It is ropey, stringy, slick, gummy, golden brown feces. When this happens, it means you are getting rid of the main culprit.

Chapter 3
Make a plan

The Number One Thing you need to do is get your head on straight. Your mind and body are not separate. Life is stressful, but don't let anything get in the way of this. If you have any excuses in your mind right now, don't start until you are ready!

You should plan to start your cleanse when you have 2 days off in a row. You will also want to begin your cleanse on your first day off. The reason is you cannot have coffee for the first 2 days. I know coffee drinkers depend on that to get them going and during these two days, Green Tea should only be consumed.

**Now for day 3 through 10: IF you can go without coffee, great! But IF you can't, coffee should be limited to 8 oz. per day. And if you are a coffee drinker that uses cream and sugar, try and do your best to avoid it for the rest of the cleanse.

The first 2 days on the cleanse, if you are **not** a diabetic, juice as much as you can!! It might be a tough 2 days, but it will be worth it! (recipes are in the back of the book)

- 2 days before you begin, you will need to drink a cup of warm water with one fresh squeezed lemon. Drink it on an empty stomach first thing in the morning. This will start cleansing your liver so it is ready to filter the toxins that are going to dislodge during your cleanse.
- Go the recipes (in "My Farmaceutical Recipes" book) and the daily routine. Decide what you will eat over the next 10 days and make a list.
- After you go shopping, wash your fruits and vegetables (make a water and vinegar bath) for the week.
- Prepare meals in advance
- If you work, put your clay and fiber in a container the night before to take to work the next day.

Look on the internet and see if there is a person who sells alkaline water that you can buy. Alkaline water will help the process because it is a restructured water. The molecules are smaller, so you will hydrate your body better. The water is also an antioxidant which will help clean your cells and the pH is usually 8.5-9.5. By drinking a high alkaline water, it raises the pH in your body, neutralizes acid and flushes toxins.

Also look for someone who does Detox Foot Baths. By having a Detox Foot Bath 1-3 times a week while you are on the cleanse, will help the body rid itself of toxins faster.

If you are unable to find either one, it's ok. They aren't necessary, they just help the process move faster.

Chapter 4
Supplements

While you are on the cleanse, I highly recommend supplements. Supplements will feed the body nutrition and help it heal while you are going through your 10 days of cleansing. Plus it can help you with the headaches, and the achiness you might experience. My choice for supplements is nutraMetrix. They offer supplements that are in powder form. There are no binders, fillers or dyes. And the absorption rate is faster because you add it to water and drink. I suggest everyone get the 90 day "Daily Essentials". They come with a Multi-Vitamin, Calcium, B Complex and OPC-3. OPC-3 is a high powered anti-oxidant and is up to 20 times more powerful than vitamin C and 50 times more powerful than vitamin E in neutralizing free radicals. *("Free radicals" is a term often used to describe damaged cells that can be problematic. They are "free" because they are missing a critical molecule, which sends them on a rampage to pair with another molecule. "These molecules will rob any molecule to quench that need," Jeffrey Blumberg, PhD, professor of nutrition at Tufts University in Boston, says.)*

If you choose nutraMetrix, it is recommended you take a cap full of each every day. When I say a cap full, I mean the cap that screws onto the bottle, use that to measure.

For pain, headaches, or extra energy take 1 cap of Calcium and 2 caps of B Complex when needed.

nutraMetrix also offers a Digestive Kit that has Aloe Juice, Digestive Enzymes and probiotics. Having these products on hand can help with possible stomach upset and to help put good bacteria back in the gut. It can also help move your bowel a little faster if it is being sluggish.

To order these products go to www.thebodymendercleanse.com

Chapter 5
When 10 Days are completed

After you have completed your 10 days, the way to tell if your colon is clean is, when you wipe and there isn't hardly anything on the paper, you know you have a clean colon. If you think you haven't completely cleaned out your colon, then continue for another 10 days. You should **NOT** do this cleanse for more than 30 days.

Every "Body" is different. Your bowel might move faster than someone elses. Please note that if you are feeling bloated or over full, drink more water. Water will help hydrate the substance in your intestines and bowel so it can move easier. Give your body a little time for your bowel to start moving.

When you have completed your cleanse, you can continue to take the fiber shake every day to keep your intestines and colon moving properly.

To reorder your products, please call 704-965-9156, or you can go to www.thebodymendercleanse.com to order online.

If you have any questions, you can either call the number above or email us info@thebodymendercleanse.com.

Chapter 6

Routine Cleanse

The intake of water during this cleanse is **VERY IMPORTANT!!!** ½ of your body weight in ounces EVERY DAY!! I have not added water to this routine because it needs to be a constant thing ALL DAY LONG and for the rest of your life!

This routine should be followed for 10 days. You can go longer if you feel it is necessary. The 10 days cleanse should be done every 6 months to keep your body functioning properly.

Breakfast

First thing in the morning, drink hot water with lemon

The reason for this is to help the liver process the particles that the colon will be releasing.

Next, make and drink the Fiber Shake

You want to drink this on an empty stomach and even though you have just drank your stomach is empty.

30 minutes later take your supplements and /or medication

It is important to wait 30 minutes after you drink the shake. The reason is, you don't want the shake to push your supplements and/or medication out of your body.

10-20 minutes later choose either Fresh Juice, Protein Shake or Eggs.

**you aren't going to want much. The Shake will fill you up. Don't over eat, but make sure you get protein.

Mid-Morning: Fiber Shake

Make sure to drink on an empty stomach

Lunch

Choose from the following

Healthy Soup and Salad
A Bean Dish
A Main Course Salad
Broiled Fish or Baked Chicken with Greens
Healthy Turkey Burger (NO BUN)

Afternoon: Fiber Shake

Make sure to drink on an empty stomach

Dinner

Choose from the following:

A Main Course Salad
Steamed Vegetables and Brown Rice
Baked Fish, Turkey or Chicken
Hearty Soup and Salad
Vegetarian Entrée with salad

An hour before bed – Herbal Tea such as Peppermint or Chamomile

Snacks that are allowed:
Raw nuts, seeds, vegetables
Fresh Vegetable Juice
Fresh Fruit
Smoothie

Beverages:
Hot Lemon Water
Iced or hot herbal tea
Water infused with fruit or cucumber

***Easy recipes that go with this Cleanse
Routine can be found in "My Farmaceutial

Recipes" by Sylvia Anton. To order your copy,
to go www.thebodymendercleanse.com

Chapter 7
Liquid Recipes

The Fiber Shake

This is a detox drink designed to remove toxins from your gut. The fiber supplement gets your digestive system moving and scrapes clean the walls of your gut, while the super-absorbent bentonite clay sucks up any toxins sitting in your intestines and carries them safely out of your body.

For the fiber supplement, you will use Colon Care Formula– it promotes colon health with fiber, calcium, magnesium, selenium and FOS probiotic growth complex. These nutrients provide dietary support for normal, healthy functioning of the colon, including regular elimination of toxins and waste material, promoting the growth of friendly bacteria, such as acidophilus and bifidus, and support for proper digestion. If you would like a little more intense cleanse, Psyllium husk is very effective, but can be quite harsh on the intestines. If you have Diabetes, extra Psyllium husk is not suggested.

Add the Bentonite Clay to your fiber supplement and shake up the mixture for a few seconds, then quickly drink it before it settles. Drink another extra-large glass of water immediately after. Both these ingredients are great for detox. The Bentonite clay soaks up toxins, and the fiber pushes waste matter out through your colon.

If you are someone who has taste or texture issues, try substituting the water with either Orange, Apple or Cranberry juice
Recipe:

4-6 oz. of water or juice
1 Tbsp. fiber supplement
1 Tbsp. liquid Bentonite Clay

Juice Recipes

The following juice recipes should not be consumed by people who have diabetes.

Holley's Favorite for Detox and Inflammation

1 peeled Cucumber
3 carrots
3 Celery sticks
1 Beet with leaves
1 cored Apple
1 Orange or Lemon (depending on your taste)

Green Drink

16 kale leaves (Tuscan cabbage)
2 cucumbers
8 celery sticks
4 apples (should use green, but whatever works for you)
1 lemon (or orange if you need a little sweetness)
2 in piece of fresh root ginger

Directions

1) Juice all the ingredients except for the avocado
2) De-seed the avocado and separate the meat from the skin
3) Blend the juice and avocado well and serve

Avocado Special

Ingredients

2 Apples
1 Avocado
3 Celery Sticks
15 Grapes
1 Lime
2 cups Spinach

A blender is required to add the avocado in since an avocado isn't very juice friendly. If you have a centrifuge juicer, I suggest blending the spinach as well since you won't get much juice out of the spinach with that kind of juicer.

You can, of course, not bother with the avocado and it'll still be delicious.

Smoothie Recipes

Green Yummy

Ingredients:
1/2 cup coconut water
4 – 6 kales leaves (Tuscan cabbage leaves)
2 celery stalks
1 zucchini
1 cucumber
4 strawberries
1/2 cup blueberries
1 handful of ice

Directions:
1. Wash all produce.
2. Juice the kale, celery, zucchini and cucumber.
3. Add the green juice and the remaining ingredients into the blender.
4. Blend until smooth and enjoy!

Substitutions:
Kale – spinach, lettuce
Celery – extra zucchini, cucumber
Zucchini – extra celery, cucumber
Cucumber – extra celery, zucchini
Strawberries – cherries, raspberries, blackberries
Blueberries – cherries, raspberries, blackberries

Blue Yummy

Ingredients:
1 cup frozen blueberries (or fresh blueberries and ice)
1/2 tsp chia seeds
14 oz. almond milk
1/2 tbsp. coconut oil
3 dates
1 tbsp. almond butter

Directions:
Add all ingredients into a blender and blend until smooth (approx. 60 – 90 seconds).

Italian Yummy

Ingredients:
12 fresh or frozen strawberries
1/2 avocado
2 tbsp. coconut flakes or fresh coconut flesh
1 1/2 cups unsweetened almond milk (substitute coconut, rice, or hemp milk of your choice)
1/2 banana

Directions:
Add all ingredients in a high-powered blender and blend on high for 45 – 60 seconds until smooth.

Yellow, White and Green

Ingredients:
2 handfuls of fresh spinach
3 romaine leaves (cos)
1 cup coconut water
1 cup pineapple
½ of a banana
Handful of ice
Squeeze of fresh lemon wedge

Directions:
Combine all ingredients into a high powered blender and blend until smooth, about 45 – 60 seconds.